Copyright 2023

All right reserved. No part of this book should be resproduce without express permission of the author.

Table of Contents

Schizophrenia is a chronic, severe mental disorder that affects the way a person thinks, acts, expresses emotions, perceives reality, and relates to others. Though schizophrenia isn't as common as other major mental illnesses, it can be the most chronic and disabling.

People with schizophrenia often have problems doing well in society, at work, at school, and in relationships. They might feel frightened and withdrawn, and could appear to have lost touch with reality. This lifelong disease can't be cured but can be controlled with proper treatment.

Contrary to popular belief, schizophrenia is not a split or multiple personality. Schizophrenia involves a psychosis, a type of mental illness in which a person can't tell what's real from what's imagined. At times, people with psychotic disorders lose touch with reality. The world may seem like a jumble of confusing thoughts, images, and sounds. Their behavior may be very strange and even shocking. A sudden change in personality and behavior, which happens when people who have it lose touch with reality, is called a psychotic episode.

BREAKFAST

1. Broccoli Cheddar Soup

Prep Time: 10 Minutes

Cook Time: 30 minutes

Servings: 4

Ingredient

- 1/4 cup unsalted butter, melted
- 1/2 white onion, diced
- 3 tablespoons all-purpose flour
- 1 cup heavy cream
- 2 1/2 cups chicken broth
- 1/2 pound broccoli florets, cut into bite size
- 1 cup carrot, julienned
- 2 cups shredded cheddar cheese
- Salt, to taste
- Ground black pepper, to taste
- Paprika, optional

Instructions

1. Heat a soup pot on medium-high heat. Melt the butter in the pot, add diced onion and sauté for 2 minutes until lightly browned and aromatic. Add all-purpose flour, cook and stir for 1 to 2 minutes.
2. Whisk in heavy cream and chicken broth. Constantly stir the soup with a wooden spoon to avoid the flour sticking to the bottom.
3. Add broccoli and carrots, and bring the soup to a simmer. Continue cooking the soup over low heat for 15 to 20 minutes until the broccoli and carrots are softened and cooked through.
4. Season the soup with salt and ground black pepper. Blend half of the soup until smooth, then pour it back into the rest. Add cheddar cheese and keep stirring until it melts.
5. Serve immediately with more cheddar cheese and paprika on top if desired.

Prep Time: 10 Minutes

Cook Time: 15 minutes

Servings: 40

Ingredient

- 1 1/2 cups all-purpose flour
- 1 teaspoon baking soda
- 1 teaspoon ground cinnamon
- 1/2 cup unsalted butter, softened
- 3/4 cup light brown sugar
- 1/4 cup white sugar
- 2 large eggs
- 1 teaspoon vanilla extract
- 3 cups Quaker oats
- 1 1/2 cups dried cranberries
- 1 cup white chocolate chips

Instructions

1. Preheat oven to 356°F (180°C).

2. Combine all-purpose flour, baking soda and ground cinnamon in a bowl, whisk well and set aside.

3. Add unsalted butter, light brown sugar and white sugar in a stand mixer with a paddle attachment. Beat all ingredients on medium speed until creamy. Add eggs, one at a time. Keep beating the mixture until the eggs are well combined about 2 minutes. Stop the mixer and scrape down the mixture with a silicone spatula, add vanilla extract and mix well.

4. Lower the speed and add in the flour mixture. Continue mixing for 2 minutes until well combined and no powder remains.

5. Fold in oats, dried cranberries and white chocolate chips.

6. Transfer the dough onto a baking sheet lined with parchment paper. Scoop 1 tablespoon of the batter, and roll it into a ball. Place each dough on the baking sheet, about 1 inch apart.

7. Bake 9 to 10 minutes for chewy cookies or 12 to 15 minutes for crispy cookies. Transfer the cookies onto a cooling rack, and let them cool completely. Sever immediately.

Prep Time: 10 Minutes

Cook Time: 45 minutes

Servings: 4

Ingredient

- 3 cups frozen corn (or 4 large ears of corn)
- 1 tablespoon extra-virgin olive oil
- 2 tablespoons salt, divided
- Ground black pepper, to taste
- 1/4 teaspoon paprika
- 1/2 white onion, sliced
- 1 1/2 tablespoons unsalted butter
- 3 cups water
- 1 cup milk (2% less fat milk or whole milk)
- 1 cup heavy (whipping) cream
- 1 sprig parsley, chopped, for garnish
- 1 tablespoon heavy (whipping) cream, for garnish

Instructions

1. Preheat the oven to 450°F (230°C).

2. Toss the frozen corn with olive oil, salt, ground black pepper and paprika. Arrange the corn in a single layer on the baking pan lined with parchment paper. Evenly smooth out the corn on the pan and bake for 15 minutes until aromatic. Remove from the oven, and set it aside.

3. Meanwhile, heat a heavy-bottomed pot (soup pot) over medium heat. Melt butter in the pot, and add onion and a pinch of salt. Sautee onion for 3 to 5 minutes until aromatic and translucent.

4. Reserve one cup of roasted corn for serving. Add the rest of the roasted corn and water. Gently stir and bring to a boil. Reduce the heat to medium-low, cover and let it simmer for 15 minutes.

5. Pureeing the soup with a blender (or an immersion blender) on high speed for 1 to 2 minutes until smooth and creamy. (Cool down the soup a little before pouring it into a blender, it helps to prevent major splashes after blending from the heat).

6. Once pureed, strain the soup through a fine-mesh sieve for a smoother texture. Return the soup to the pot and add milk and heavy cream. Simmer the soup for 10 to 15 minutes over low heat, constantly stirring it to avoid sticking to the bottom. Add salt and ground black pepper to taste.

7. For serving, add one cup of roasted corn to the soup. Stir well and serve it either hot or chilled with freshly chopped parsley and heavy cream drizzled on top.

Prep Time: 10 Minutes

Cook Time: 5 minutes

Servings: 3

Ingredient

- 12 oz. 340 g salmon, cut into 2-3 fillet strips
- Salt
- Black pepper
- 1 pinch cayenne pepper
- 2 tablespoons honey
- 1 tablespoon warm water
- 1 1/2 teaspoons apple cider vinegar or lemon juice
- 1 tablespoon olive oil
- 3 cloves garlic minced
- 1/2 lemon sliced into wedges
- 1 tablespoon chopped parsley

Instructions

1. Season the surface of the salmon with salt, black pepper and cayenne pepper. Set aside.

2. Mix the honey, water, apple cider vinegar or lemon juice and a pinch of salt together. Stir to combine well.

3. Heat up an oven-safe skillet (cast-iron skillet preferred) on high heat. Add the olive oil. Pan-fry the salmon, skin side down first, for about 1 minute. Turn the salmon over and cook for 1 minute. Turn it over again so the skin side is at the bottom.

4. Add the garlic into the pan, sauté until slightly browned. Add the honey mixture and lemon wedges into the skillet, reduce the sauce until it's sticky.

5. Salmon with honey garlic sauce is one of the best salmon recipes.

6. Finish it off by broiling the salmon in the oven for 1 minute or until the surface becomes slightly charred (optional step).

7. Top the salmon with parsley and serve immediately.

Prep Time: 5 Minutes

Cook Time: 10 minutes

Servings: 2

Ingredient

- 1 lb. (0.4 kg) cod fillets, rinsed and pat dry
- 1/4 teaspoon salt
- 1 tablespoon lemon juice, freshly squeezed
- 3 dashes cayenne pepper
- 1 1/2 tablespoons olive oil
- 1 tablespoon chopped parsley

Instructions

1. Preheat oven to 400°F (207°C).
2. Arrange the cod fillets in baking tray. Drizzle the olive oil onto the fish, follow by lemon juice, salt and cayenne pepper.
3. Bake the cod in the oven for 10 - 12 minutes, depends on the thickness of the cod. Garnish with parsley and serve immediately.

Prep Time: 3 Minutes

Cook Time: 12 minutes

Servings: 3

Ingredient

- 15 oz. 430 g center cut boneless pork chops (3 pork chops)
- Salt
- Ground black pepper
- 1 tablespoon vegetable oil
- 2 tablespoon unsalted butter melted
- 3 cloves garlic minced
- 1 teaspoon chopped Italian parsley for garnishing

Honey Sauce:

- 2 1/2 tablespoons honey
- 2 tablespoons warm water
- 1/4 teaspoon salt
- 1/2 teaspoon apple cider vinegar
- 3 dashes cayenne pepper

Instruction

1. Season the pork chops with salt and ground black pepper, on both sides of the pork. Mix all the ingredients in the Honey Garlic Sauce together. Stir to combine well.
2. Boneless pork chops
3. Heat up a cast-iron skillet (preferred) on high heat. Add the vegetable oil and 1 tablespoon of the butter.
4. Boneless pork chops
5. Add the pork chops to the skillet and pan fry each side of the pork, uninterrupted, for 3-4 minutes each, or until the surface turns brown. Flip over to the other side and repeat the same.
6. Push the pork chops to one side of the skillet, add the remaining butter. Add the garlic and sauté for 10 seconds, or until they turn light brown. Add the Honey Garlic Sauce, cook to reduce the sauce to a thicker consistency or until the sauce turns amber brown.
7. Boneless pork chops
8. Spoon the sauce over the pork chops. Turn off the heat, garnish with the parsley and serve immediately.

Prep Time: 5 Minutes

Cook Time: 10 minutes

Servings: 3

Ingredient

- 1 lb. 0.4 kg chicken tenders
- 1 teaspoon smoked paprika
- 3 dashes cayenne powder
- 4 tablespoons unsalted butter room temperature
- 3 - 4 cloves garlic minced
- 1 teaspoon bottled Italian seasoning Simply Organic or McCormick brand
- Salt to taste
- 1/2 tablespoon lemon juice
- 1 tablespoon chopped parsley
- Lemon wedges

Instructions

1. Season the chicken tenders with smoked paprika and cayenne pepper. Set aside.

2. Chicken tenders.

3. Heat up a cast-iron skillet (preferred) on high heat and add 3 tablespoons of butter. As soon as the butter melts and starts to sizzle, add the chicken tenders. Cook uninterrupted for 1-2 minutes, then turn over and start cooking the other side.

4. Push the chicken tenders to the side of the skillet. Add the remaining 1 tablespoon of butter follow by the minced garlic on the empty space on the skillet. Add the Italian seasoning on top of the chicken tenders and stir to combine well with the chicken and garlic.

5. Add salt and lemon juice and continue to cook the chicken tenders until they are slightly charred on the both sides. Add the chopped parsley, stir to combine well. Turn off the heat and serve immediately with lemon wedges. Squeeze the lemon juice on top before serving.

Prep Time: 10 Minutes

Cook Time: 3hrs 30 minutes

Servings: 3

Ingredient

- 1 1/2 lbs. 0.6 kg chicken wings, drumettes and mid sections
- 1 inch 2 cm piece ginger, peeled and sliced
- 1 tablespoon soy sauce
- 1 tablespoon oyster sauce
- 2 tablespoons honey
- 1 tablespoon cooking sake or rice wine optional
- 3 dashes ground white pepper
- 1/2 tablespoon sesame oil
- 1/2 tablespoon dark soy sauce for coloring purpose (optional)
- 1/2 tablespoon corn starch plus 2 tablespoons water
- Salt to taste
- White sesame seeds for garnishing

Instructions

1. Rinse the chicken wings with cold water, drained.
2. Transfer the chicken wings and all the ingredients into a slow cooker. Stir to combine well.
3. Cook on high heat for 3 1/2 hours. Turn off the heat, dish out, top with some white sesame, and serve immediately.

Prep Time: 15 Minutes

Cook Time: 4hrs 5 minutes

Servings: 6

Ingredient

- 2 1/2 pounds 1125 g pork roast, diced into 6 pieces
- 1/2 white onion diced
- 4 cloves garlic smashed with the side of a knife and peeled
- 1/4 cup 60 ml soy sauce
- 1/4 cup 45 g dark brown sugar
- 2 tablespoons 30 ml honey
- 1 tablespoon 11 g sesame seeds
- 1 tablespoon 15 g corn starch
- 3 Thai chili peppers sliced

Instruction

1. In a crock pot, add the pork roast, onion, garlic, soy sauce, brown sugar, honey and sesame seeds; stir until

the pork is coated with the other ingredients. Cook on high for 4 hours.

2. Transfer the pork to a cutting board and shred using two forks.

3. In a pot, add the reserved juices from the crock pot and whisk in the corn starch. Cook on medium-high heat until the sauce thickens. Stir in the chili peppers and shredded pork.

4. Serve the pork over steamed white rice.

Prep Time: 10 Minutes

Cook Time: 4hrs 30 minutes

Servings: 4

Ingredient

- 2 boneless chicken breasts
- 1/8 cup dry sake
- 1/8 cup miring
- 1/4 cup soy sauce
- 3 tablespoons honey
- 2 cloves garlic minced
- 2 tablespoons ginger minced
- Freshly ground black pepper
- 1/8 cup water
- 1 1/2 tablespoons corn starch
- 2 stalks green onions chopped
- Toasted sesame seeds

Instructions

1. In a crockpot, combine the chicken, sake, miring, soy sauce, honey, garlic and ginger. Season with black pepper, to taste. Turn on the crockpot to high and cook for 4 to 4 1/2 hours.
2. Transfer the chicken to a cutting board and shred using two forks.
3. Pour the reserved liquid from the crock pot into a small sauce pot and heat to a rolling boil. Mix together the water and corn starch; stir it into the sauce and cook until thick. Add the chicken to the pot, and top with sesame seeds and green onions.

11. Crock Pot Asian Beef Stew

Prep Time: 10 Minutes

Cook Time: 8hrs 3 minutes

Servings: 4

Ingredient

- 1 yellow onion diced
- 4 cloves garlic minced
- 1 tablespoon 10 g ginger, peeled and sliced
- 1 cup 150 g mini carrots
- 1/2 pound 230 g bottom eye roast or bottom round roast, diced into 1" cubes
- 2 tablespoons 30 ml soy sauce
- 2 tablespoons 30 ml oyster sauce
- 1 teaspoon 5 ml sesame oil
- 1 tablespoon Chinese rice wine (15 mL)
- 1 cup 240 ml water
- Black pepper to taste
- 1 tablespoon chopped green onions

Instructions

1. In a crock pot, add all the ingredients in the listed order for the exception of the green onions.
2. Turn the crock pot on low and allow the stew to cook for 8 hours. Halfway through the cook time, stir the ingredients to evenly season the ingredients.
3. Serve over white rice and top with green onions, if using.

Prep Time: 15 Minutes

Cook Time: 15 minutes

Servings: 4

Ingredient

- 1 lb. 0.4 kg boneless and skinless chicken breasts, pat dry and cut into cubes
- Salt
- Ground black pepper
- 2 large eggs beaten
- 1 cup panko or breadcrumbs
- White sesame seeds for garnishing
- Chopped scallions or chives for garnishing

Honey Garlic Sauce:

- 2 cloves garlic finely minced
- 4 tablespoons honey
- 2 tablespoons soy sauce
- 2 tablespoons Thai sweet chili sauce
- 1/4 cup water
- 1/2 tablespoon corn starch

Instructions

1. Preheat the oven to 375°F (190°C).

2. Season the chicken with salt and black pepper. Coat each piece of the chicken with the beaten eggs first, then roll in the panko. Repeat to nicely coat the chicken.

3. Transfer the chicken to a baking sheet lined with parchment paper. Bake for about 12-15 minutes, or until the chicken turn golden brown. You might turn the chicken pieces over to bake the other side.

4. Mix all the ingredients for the Sauce in a small sauce. Whisk to mix well. Cook on low heat until the sauce slightly thickens.

5. Transfer the chicken out into a bowl and add the Sauce mixture. Gently toss to coat well. Garnish with the white sesame and scallions/chives, serve immediately.

Prep Time: 5 Minutes

Cook Time: 40 minutes

Servings: 3

Ingredient

- 1 1/2 lbs. 0.5 kg chicken thighs
- 1 2 inch 5 cm piece ginger, peeled and chopped
- 3 cloves garlic peeled and chopped
- 1 tablespoon soy sauce
- 1 tablespoon oyster sauce
- 1 tablespoon honey
- 1 teaspoon sesame oil
- 3 dashes white pepper
- 1 pinch salt

Instructions

1. Rinse the chicken thighs and pat dry with paper towels. Add the ginger and garlic to the chicken and gently rub them on the chicken thighs. Add the rest of the ingredients to the chicken thighs, stir to coat well.

2. Set aside to marinate for at least 30 minutes.

3. Pre-heat the oven to 375°F (190°C). Line the chicken on a tray lined with aluminium foil and bake for 40 minutes in the middle of the oven.

4. Or until the surface turn golden brown, slightly charred and the inside of the chicken thighs are cooked. Serve immediately.

Prep Time: 35 Minutes

Cook Time: 25 minutes

Servings: 2

Ingredient

- 2 tablespoons all-purpose flour plus more for surface
- 1 package about 1 pound frozen puff pastry preferably all butter, thawed
- 2 tablespoons unsalted butter
- 1/2 1 cup onion, diced
- 1 1/3 cup small carrot, peeled and thinly sliced
- 1 1/3 cup stalk thinly sliced celery
- 1 small Yukon Gold potato scrubbed and cut into a 1/2-inch dice
- 1 1/4 cups low-sodium chicken broth
- 1 cup 2 oz. packed coarsely chopped collard-green leaves
- 8 oz. 226 g boneless, skinless chicken breast, cut into 1-inch chunks
- Coarse salt and freshly ground pepper
- 1 large egg lightly beaten

Instructions

1. Preheat oven to 425°F (217°C). Place a 1 1/2-cup ovenproof dish on pastry on a floured surface. Cut a circle from pastry, 1/2 inch larger than dish; cut vents. Repeat. Refrigerate on a parchment-lined baking sheet.

2. Melt butter in a large skillet over medium heat. Add onion. Cook, stirring, until soft, 4 minutes. Add carrot, celery, and potato. Cook, stirring, until soft, 6 minutes. Stir in flour, then broth; bring to a boil. Add greens and chicken. Simmer until thickened, 2 minutes; season.

3. Divide between dishes. Top with pastry, press edges to seal, and brush with egg. Bake on a baking sheet until golden, 25 minutes.

Prep Time: 20 Minutes

Cook Time: 10 minutes

Servings: 3

Ingredient

- 3 chicken thighs deboned, and cut into halves
- 2 cloves garlic minced
- 1/2 teaspoon five-spice powder
- 1/2 teaspoon sesame oil
- 1 teaspoon Chinese rice wine or Japanese cooking sake optional
- 1 teaspoon oyster sauce
- 1 teaspoon soy sauce
- 1 teaspoon sugar
- Salt to taste
- 1/2 tablespoon oil

Instructions

1. Deboned the chicken thighs and keep the skin. You may use skinless and boneless chicken thighs, too.

2. Marinate the chicken with garlic, five spice powder, sesame oil, rice wine, oyster sauce, soy sauce, sugar and salt for 15 minutes, or best for 1 hour.

3. Add the oil in your skillet on medium heat. Pan-fry the chicken on both sides until browned and crispy, and the inside is cooked through. Dish out and serve immediately.

Prep Time: 30 Minutes

Cook Time: 40 minutes

Servings: 3

Ingredient

- 1 3/4 lbs. 800 g chicken drumsticks
- 2 tablespoons finely chopped cilantro stems
- 3 cloves garlic minced
- Chopped cilantro leaves for garnishing
- Thai sweet chili sauce for dipping

Marinade:

- 1 tablespoon oil
- 1 3/4 tablespoons fish sauce
- 2 tablespoons coconut milk
- 1 tablespoon honey or Thai palm sugar
- 3 dashes ground black pepper
- 1 pinch cayenne pepper
- 1 pinch turmeric powder

Instructions

1. Preheat oven to 375°F (190°C).

2. Rinse the chicken and pat dry with paper towels. Combine all the ingredients in Marinade, whisk to mix well to form a nice milky pale yellow mixture.

3. Add the cilantro and garlic to the chicken, rub onto the chicken drumsticks with your hand. Add the Marinade to the chicken, mix to coat well and marinate for 30 minutes or best for two hours.

4. Arrange the chicken on a cookie sheet lined with parchment paper, bake for 40 minutes or until the chicken is cooked through. Garnish with chopped cilantro and serve immediately with Thai sweet chili sauce.

Prep Time: 5 Minutes

Cook Time: 15 minutes

Servings: 4

Ingredient

- 20 oz. 600 g chicken thighs, skin-on and deboned
- 2 tablespoons olive oil
- 15-20 cloves garlic
- 1/2 cup chicken broth
- 1/3 cup white wine
- 1/4 cup plain yogurt
- 3 sprigs thyme optional
- Salt to taste
- Ground black pepper
- 1 pinch paprika
- Chopped parsley

Instructions

1. Season the chicken with a little salt and pepper.

2. Heat up a skillet (cast-iron skillet preferred) on medium heat, add 1 tablespoon of olive oil. Pan-fry the chicken until both surfaces become crispy or nicely browned. Remove the chicken from the skillet and set aside.

3. Discard the chicken fat from the skillet. Add the remaining olive oil and saute the garlic until light brown. Add the chicken back into the skillet, follow by the chicken broth, white wine and yogurt. Lower the heat and let simmer.

4. Add the thymes (if using), salt, pepper and paprika. Reduce the sauce a little bit. Remove from heat, garnish with parsley and serve immediately.

Prep Time: 10 Minutes

Cook Time: 10 minutes

Servings: 2

Ingredient

- 4-6 oz (100-175 g) beef tenderloin, cut into bite-sized pieces
- 1 lb (500 g) fresh flat rice noodles
- 2 tablespoons oil
- 2 cloves garlic, minced
- 1 cup fresh bean sprouts, ends trimmed
- 1 oz. (50g) green onion (scallion) or yellow chives, cut into 2 inches lengths

Marinade:

- 2 teaspoons soy sauce
- 1/2 teaspoon dark soy sauce
- 1/2 teaspoon Chinese rice wine or sherry
- 1 heaping teaspoon cornstarch

Seasonings:

- 2 1/2 tablespoons soy sauce

- 1 teaspoon dark soy sauce

- 1 tablespoon oyster sauce

- 1/2 teaspoon fish sauce

- 1/2 teaspoon sugar

Instructions

1. Add beef slices, soy sauce, dark soy sauce, Chinese rice wine, and cornstarch to a bowl, and marinate for 15 minutes.

2. Loosen the flat rice noodles completely so they don't clump together.

3. Add all seasoning ingredients to a small bowl, and mix well. Set aside.

4. Heat the oil in a wok or skillet over high heat. Add the garlic and stir-fry until light brown and aromatic. Add beef and stir-fry until they are half-cooked, and then follow with the bean sprouts, flat rice noodles, and the seasonings.

5. Toss the flat rice noodles with a spatula or chopsticks until the seasonings are well combined with the noodles. Continue stir-frying for another 1-2 minutes until the noodles are slightly charred. Finally, add the

green onion or yellow chives and stir-fry for another 10 seconds.

6. Turn off the heat and transfer the beef chow fun noodles to a serving platter. Serve immediately.

Prep Time: 5 Minutes

Cook Time: 10 minutes

Servings: 4

Ingredient

- 2 tablespoons corn starch
- 3 tablespoons water
- 1 3/4 cups chicken broth
- 1 1/2 cups water
- 6 oz chicken breast (or ground chicken, chicken thigh), skinless, cut into bite-size pieces
- 1 can creamy sweet corn
- 3 dashes white pepper
- 1/2 teaspoon salt
- 2 eggs, beaten
- Cilantro, to garnish

Instructions

1. Mix corn starch and water in a small bowl; stir well and set aside.

2. Add chicken broth and water to a soup pot and bring to a boil. Lower the heat to medium and add chicken breast into the soup. (If using ground chicken, break up the chicken into small pieces with a fork before cooking.) Skim off the foam on the surface. Continue cooking the chicken for 3 to 5 minutes until cooked through.

3. Add the creamy sweet corn, white pepper, and salt and thicken the soup with cornstarch mixture. (Gently stir the cornstarch mixture before adding to the soup.) Stir the soup with a ladle and turn off the heat.

4. Swirl the beaten eggs into the soup and immediately stir a few times with a pair of chopsticks. Cover the pot with a lid for 2 minutes. The eggs should be cooked and will form into silken threads.

5. Dish out and serve immediately with cilantro leaves on top.

Prep Time: 10 Minutes

Cook Time: 10 minutes

Servings: 4

Ingredient

- 6 oz (175 g) ground beef
- 1/2 tablespoon Chinese rice wine or sherry
- 1/2 teaspoon sesame oil
- 2 1/2 tablespoons cornstarch
- 3 tablespoons water
- 1 can (14 oz/ 400 g) store-bought chicken broth
- 1 1/3 cups (375 ml) water
- 3 dashes white pepper
- 1/2 teaspoon salt to taste
- 2 large eggs, lightly beaten
- 1/2 cup (10 g) coarsely chopped coriander leaves (cilantro)

Instructions

1. Marinate the ground beef with Chinese rice wine (or sherry) and sesame oil for 10 minutes. Break up the ground beef into small pieces using a fork (or a pair of chopsticks) and stir well while marinating.
2. Mix cornstarch and 3 tablespoons of water in a small bowl; stir well and set aside.
3. Bring chicken broth and 1 1/3 cups of water to a boil in a soup pot. Lower the heat to medium and add ground beef to the soup. Skim off the foam on the surface.
4. Add white pepper and salt, and thicken the soup with the cornstarch mixture. Stir the soup with a ladle to smooth the texture and turn off the heat.
5. Swirl the beaten eggs into the soup and immediately stir it three times with a pair of chopsticks. Cover the pot with its lid for 2 minutes and the egg should be cooked with the remaining heat. Add the coriander leaves into the soup and stir to blend well.
6. Dish out and serve immediately.

21. Shrimp and Broccoli

Prep Time: 10 Minutes

Cook Time: 5 minutes

Servings: 2

Ingredient

- 1/2 lb broccoli florets
- 1/2 lb headless shrimp, shelled and deveined
- 2 tablespoons cooking oil
- 2 cloves garlic, minced
- Sauce
- 1 tablespoon soy sauce
- 1 tablespoon oyster sauce
- 1 teaspoon sesame oil
- 2 teaspoons sugar
- 1 teaspoon corn starch
- 1/4 cup cold water
- 3 dashes ground white pepper

Instructions

1. Combine all sauce ingredients in a bowl, whisk well and set aside.

2. Wash and rinse the broccoli with running water. Heat up a pot of water and bring it to a boil. Cook the broccoli florets for 1 minute and transfer them to a bowl of ice-cold water. Cool down for 5 minutes, drain and set aside.

3. Rinse and pat dry shrimp with paper towels. Heat the wok or skillet on high heat, and add the oil. When the oil is heated, add the garlic and stir-fry until aromatic or becomes light brown. Add the shrimp and stir a few times until cooked through or turned pink.

4. Turn the heat to medium-low. (Give the sauce a little bit of stir before pouring it into the wok). Add broccoli and sauce, stir continuously for 1 minute until the sauce thickens. Turn off the heat and dish out. Serve immediately.

Prep Time: 10 Minutes

Cook Time: 5 minutes

Servings: 3

Ingredient

- 3 fresh Persian cucumbers
- 3 teaspoons low-sodium soy sauce
- 5 tablespoons Chinese black vinegar
- 1 tablespoon granulated sugar
- 1 tablespoon spicy chili crisp (or chili oil)
- 1 tablespoon sesame oil
- 1/2 tablespoon roasted sesame seeds
- Salt to taste
- 2 cloves garlic, minced
- 1 stalk scallion, chopped
- 2 red Red Thai pepper, chopped
- 3 stalk cilantro, chopped

Instructions

1. Wash and slice off the ends of cucumbers on a cutting board. Place the side of the knife against the cucumber and gently smash the cucumber with your palm until it splits. Then, cut into 1/2-inch thick pieces and transfer them to a large bowl.

2. Prepare salad dressing by combining soy sauce, vinegar, sugar, spicy chili crisp, sesame oil, roasted sesame seeds, and salt in a small bowl. Stir until sugar and salt are dissolved. Set aside.

3. Top the smashed cucumber pieces with minced garlic, chopped scallion, red Thai pepper, and chopped cilantro in a large bowl. Toss well with prepared salad dressing.

4. Dish out and serve immediately.

Prep Time: 15 Minutes

Cook Time: 10 minutes

Servings: 6

Ingredient

- 2 packets active dry yeast total 1/2 oz or 14 g + 1 tablespoon sugar
- 1/4 cup warm water
- 1 1/4 cups milk
- 5 tablespoons sugar
- 3/4 teaspoon salt
- 1/4 cup 1/2 stick unsalted butter
- 4 1/2 cups sifted all-purpose flour
- 1 large egg
- Baking spray
- 1 teaspoon kosher salt
- 3 tablespoons melted unsalted butter

Instruction

1. Dissolve the yeast with the sugar in warm water. Heat the milk with the sugar, salt, butter until lukewarm.

2. Add the egg to the yeast mixture. Combine the yeast mixture, the milk mixture, and all of the flour. Stir to combine well. Cover the dough and rest for 15 minutes. Using a stand mixer with a dough hook, knead the dough for 5 minutes

3. Preheat oven to 375°F (190°C).

4. On a floured surface, roll out the dough and divide it into 18 balls, about the size of a small tennis ball. Cover and let rise for 25 minutes. Spray the baking spray on a 10-inch cast-iron skillet, arrange the dough balls on the skillet. Sprinkle the kosher salt evenly on the surface. Bake for 10-12 minutes, or until the surface of the dinner rolls turn golden brown. Brush with the melted butter and serve warm.

Prep Time: 20 Minutes

Cook Time: 10 minutes

Servings: 24

Ingredient

- 2 packets active dry yeast total 1/2 oz. or 14 g + 1 tablespoon sugar
- 1/4 cup warm water
- 1 1/4 cups milk
- 5 tablespoons sugar
- 3/4 teaspoon salt
- 1/4 cup 1/2 stick butter unsalted butter
- 4 1/2 cups sifted all-purpose flour
- 1 large egg

Toppings:

- 4 cloves garlic finely minced
- 1/2 cup salted butter melted
- 2 tablespoons chopped parsley
- 1/3 cup shredded Parmesan cheese

Instructions

1. Dissolve the yeast plus 1 tablespoon of sugar in warm water. Then heat the milk with the sugar, salt, butter until lukewarm.

2. Add the egg to the yeast mixture. Combine the yeast mixture, the milk mixture, and all of the flour. Stir to combine well. Cover the dough and rest for 15 minutes. Using a stand mixer with a dough hook, knead the dough for 5 minutes.

3. Preheat oven to 350°F (176°C).

4. On a floured surface, roll out the dough and divide it into 24 balls. Roll out each ball and tie each into a knot. Cover and let rise for 25 minutes.

5. Garlic Parmesan Dinner Rolls

6. Meanwhile, prepare the garlic-herb butter by combining all the Toppings ingredients together, except Parmesan cheese. Brush the butter mixture generously on the surface and top with Parmesan cheese.

7. Bake for 10-15 minutes, or until in the middle of the dinner rolls are cooked through and the tops turn golden brown. Brush with the remaining butter mixture and serve warm.

Prep Time: 25 Minutes

Cook Time: 15 minutes

Servings: 24

Ingredient

- 2 1/2 teaspoons instant yeast
- 1/4 cup brown sugar
- 1/2 cup lukewarm milk
- 4 tablespoons softened butter
- 2 teaspoons salt
- 2 teaspoons pumpkin pie spice
- 2 large eggs
- 3/4 cup pumpkin purée canned pumpkin
- 4 cups all-purpose flour

Instructions

1. Combine all of the ingredients in a large bowl, mix and knead — using your hands, a stand mixer, or a bread machine set on the dough cycle — to make a soft, smooth dough.

2. Place the dough in a lightly greased bowl, and allow it to rise for 60 to 75 minutes, until it's puffy though not necessarily doubled in bulk. Gently deflate the dough, and transfer it to a lightly greased work surface. Divide the dough into 24 equal pieces. Round each piece into a smooth ball.

3. Lightly grease a large cast-iron skillet or a sheet pan and arrange the dough. Cover the skillet or sheet pan, and allow the rolls to rise until they're crowded against one another and quite puffy, about 1 1/2 to 2 hours. Towards the end of the rising time, preheat the oven to 350°F (176°C).

4. Uncover the rolls, and bake them for about 20 minutes. Cover the top with aluminum foil if they brown too fast. Remove the rolls from the oven, and brush with melted butter. Serve warm. Freeze for longer storage.

Prep Time: 10 Minutes

Cook Time: 35 minutes

Servings: 6

Ingredient

- 4 tablespoons unsalted butter
- 2 tablespoons olive oil
- 4 cups yellow onion, sliced
- 5 cups beef broth
- 2 tablespoons dry sherry
- 1 teaspoon dried thyme
- Salt, to taste
- Ground black pepper, to taste
- 6 slices French bread
- 6 slices Provolone cheese
- 4 slices Swiss cheese, diced
- 1/4 cup grated Parmesan cheese

Instructions

1. Heat the dutch oven or a large pot on medium heat. Add butter and olive oil, keep stirring until the butter melts.
2. Add onion slices and occasionally stir until soft and translucent. It takes about 8 to 10 minutes.
3. Add beef broth, dry sherry and dried thyme. Season the soup with salt and ground black pepper, and stir well. Simmer the soup for 30 minutes over medium heat.
4. Preheat broiler to high.
5. Ladle soup into oven-safe ramekins and top each with one slice of French bread, a slice of provolone cheese, a couple of diced swish cheese and finish with more grated parmesan cheese on top.
6. Broil for 2 to 3 minutes until golden brown on the edges.
7. Serve immediately with freshly chopped parsley on top.

Prep Time: 5 Minutes

Cook Time: 20 minutes

Servings: 4

Ingredient

- 1/4 cup unsalted butter
- 3 red apples, unpeeled and thinly sliced
- 3/4 cup white sugar, divided
- 1/2 teaspoon ground cinnamon
- Vanilla ice cream, for serving

Instructions

1. Melt the butter in a medium dutch oven or a cast-iron skillet on medium heat. Add apple slices and 1/2 cup of the sugar, stir well.
2. Bring to a simmer, cover and cook on medium-low heat for 15 minutes until the apples are softened. Stir occasionally to prevent the apples from sticking to the bottom.

3. Add the remaining sugar and cinnamon, stir constantly and cook for another 5 to 10 minutes over medium-high heat.

4. Serve immediately with ice cream or as a topping for waffles or pancakes.

Prep Time: 5 Minutes

Cook Time: 40 minutes

Servings: 4

Ingredient

- 4 cups water
- 1 sheet dried kelp
- 8 dried anchovies
- 2 tablespoons oil
- 1 yellow onion, sliced
- 4 cloves garlic, minced
- 1 cup kimchee, chopped (more kimchee juice to taste)
- 1/2 lb pork belly, cut into bite size pieces
- 3 stalks green onion, sliced into 2-inch pieces
- 1 tablespoon gochugaru powder (Korean hot pepper flakes)
- 1 tablespoon gochujang (Korean red chili paste)
- 1 tablespoon sesame oil
- 1 teaspoon soy sauce
- 1/2 teaspoon sugar
- 1 pack of firm tofu

- Salt, to taste
- Ground black pepper, to taste

Instructions

1. Prepare the anchovy kelp stock. Remove the heads and guts from the dried anchovies first. Bring water to a boil in a saucepan then add dried anchovies and kelp. Cover and cook the soup over medium heat. Continue simmering for 15 minutes. Turn off the heat, strain the broth into a bowl and remove the solids. Set aside.

2. Heat a soup pot (or a Korean earthenware pot) with oil on medium-high heat. Add onion and garlic and stir-fry for 2 minutes until aromatic.

3. Add kimchee, 2 tablespoons of kimchee juice, and pork belly. Stir constantly for 5 minutes until the meat is almost cooked through.

4. In a small bowl, combine green onion, gochugaru powder, gochujang, sesame oil, soy sauce and sugar. Mix well. Stir into the pot.

5. Add anchovy kelp stock and bring the soup to a boil. Then, lower the heat to medium-low and simmer for 10 to 15 minutes.

6. Cut the tofu in half lengthwise and slice into 1-inch pieces. Add tofu, and simmer for 10 minutes until the tofu soaked with all the flavor from the stew and the pork is cooked through.

7. Serve immediately with chopped green onion garnish on top.

Prep Time: 10 Minutes

Cook Time: 20 minutes

Servings: 4

Ingredient

- 1/2 lb sirloin steak, diced
- 1/2 lb shrimp, peeled and deveined
- 2 ears corn, chopped into 3 equal pieces
- 4 cherry tomatoes, cut into wedges
- 1 small red onion, thinly sliced
- 2 limes cut in wedges
- 4 cloves garlic, sliced
- 2 tablespoons Old Bay seasoning
- 1 tablespoon fresh thyme leaves
- 1 teaspoon ground cumin
- 1 teaspoon ground black pepper
- Olive oil, to drizzle on top
- 1 tablespoon fresh parsley, chopped, for garnish

Instructions

1. Prepare four 12-inch long aluminum foil sheets.

2. Dice the steak into 1-inch thick cubes and cut each ear of corn into 3 equal pieces.

3. Divide steak, shrimp, corn, tomato wedges, red onion slices, lime wedges, and garlic slices on each piece of foil. Sprinkle with Old Bay seasoning, fresh thyme leaves, ground cumin, and ground black pepper and drizzle olive oil on top.

4. Fold the foil in half and roll up the edges to seal the food tightly inside.

5. Heat the grill to high. Place the foil packs on the grill and cook for 8 to 10 minutes per side. Remove the packs from the grill once the shrimp is cooked through and the steak is cooked to your desired doneness.

6. Serve immediately with freshly chopped parsley on top and lime wedges. Sprinkle more Old Bay seasoning for serving if desired.

Prep Time: 10 Minutes

Cook Time: 20 minutes

Servings: 5

Ingredient

- 1 1/2 lb boneless skinless chicken breast
- 5 tablespoons olive oil, divided
- Juice of 1 lemon, divided
- Salt, to taste
- Ground black pepper, to taste
- 1 teaspoon Italian seasoning
- 3 vine-ripened tomatoes, diced
- 2 cloves garlic, minced
- 1 tablespoon freshly chopped basil
- 4 slices of mozzarella cheese
- Grated parmesan cheese, for serving

1. Rinse and pat dry chicken breast with kitchen paper towels. Cut chicken breast into four to five equal parts. Transfer to a large bowl and set aside.

2. Add 4 tablespoons of olive oil, 1/2 lemon juice, salt, ground black pepper and Italian seasoning in a small bowl, whisk to combine. Then, pour into the large bowl and marinate the chicken breast for 30 minutes in the refrigerator.

3. Heat a cast-iron skillet on high heat and add 1 tablespoon of olive oil. Place the marinated chicken breast on the skillet and cook for 8 to 10 minutes on each side until charred. (You may cook 2 to 3 minutes longer if the meat is large and thick.)

4. Meanwhile, prepare the tomato mixture in a small bowl. Add diced tomatoes, minced garlic, chopped basil, and the remaining lemon juice to the bowl. Add salt and ground black pepper and toss well.

5. Top each chicken breast with a slice of mozzarella cheese and continue cooking for 2 to 3 minutes until the cheese is melted.

6. Dish out. Add a spoonful of the tomato mixture to each chicken breast and top with grated parmesan cheese. Serve immediatel